COMPLETE GUIDE TO OVARIAN CYSTECTOMY

Essential Handbook To Expert Techniques, Minimally Invasive Procedures, Recovery Tips, And Patient Care

DR. BRUNO HORAN

Copyright © 2023 by Dr. Bruno Horan

All rights reserved. Except for brief quotations embodied in critical reviews and certain other noncommercial uses permitted by copyright law, no part of this publication may be reproduced, distributed, or transmitted in any form or by any means, Including photocopying, recording, or other electronic or mechanical methods, without the prior written permission of the publisher.

Disclaimer:

The information provided in this book, is intended for general informational purposes only and should not be considered as professional advice.

The author has made every effort to ensure the accuracy of the information presented. However, readers are advised to consult with a qualified healthcare professional before attempting any herbal remedies or making significant changes to their wellness routine. Individual health conditions vary, and what may be suitable for one person may not be appropriate for another.

It is important to note that the author is not in any endorsement deal, partnership, or affiliation with any organization, brand, or company mentioned in this book. Any references to specific products or services are based on the author's personal experience or general knowledge and do not imply an endorsement or promotion of those products or services

Contents

CHAPTER ONE 13
  BASICS OF OVARIAN CYSTS 13
    Types Of Ovarian Cysts 13
    Causes And Risk Factors 14
    Symptoms And Signs 14
    Diagnosis Methods 15
    Importance Of Early Detection 15

CHAPTER TWO 17
  PREPARATION FOR SURGERY 17
    Initial Consultation With Your Doctor 17
    Pre-Operative Tests And Evaluations 18
    Medications And Dietary Guidelines 18
    Psychological Preparation 19
    Preparing For Recovery At Home 20

CHAPTER THREE 21
  SURGICAL TECHNIQUES 21
    Laparoscopic Cystectomy 21
    Robotic-Assisted Cystectomy 23
    Choosing The Right Approach 24
    Benefits And Risks Of Each Technique 25

CHAPTER FOUR 27
DURING THE PROCEDURE 27
- Operating Room Setup 27
- Anesthesia Options 27
- Step-By-Step Surgical Process 28
- Role Of The Surgical Team 29
- Monitoring And Safety Measures 30

CHAPTER FIVE 31
RECOVERY AND POST-OPERATIVE CARE 31
- Immediate Post-Surgery Recovery 31
- Pain Management Strategies 32
- Diet And Activity Guidelines 32
- Follow-Up Appointments 33
- Recognizing Complications 34

CHAPTER SIX 35
COMMON CONCERNS 35
- Understanding Ovarian Cystectomy: A Comprehensive Guide 35
- Recurrence Of Ovarian Cysts 36
- Long-Term Effects Of Cystectomy 37
- Lifestyle Changes Post-Surgery 37

Emotional And Psychological Support..................38
CHAPTER SEVEN 39
FAQS (FREQUENTLY ASKED QUESTIONS) 39
How Long Does The Surgery Take? 39
When Can I Resume Normal Activities?..............39
Will My Ovarian Function Be Affected? 40
What Are The Chances Of Cyst Recurrence? 40
How Can I Prevent Future Cysts? 41
CHAPTER EIGHT 43
PATIENT STORIES AND EXPERIENCES 43
Real-Life Accounts Of Cystectomy Patients.........43
Advice And Insights From Survivors...................45
Coping Strategies Shared By Patients 46
Inspirational Stories Of Recovery.......................46
CHAPTER NINE 49
RESOURCES AND FURTHER READING...................49
Recommended Books And Articles.....................49
Online Support Groups And Forums...................50
Educational Websites..50
Contact Information For Medical Professionals....51

Additional Resources For Ongoing Support.........51

ABOUT THIS BOOK

Discover the comprehensive guide to 'Complete Guide To Ovarian Cystectomy,' an indispensable resource designed to empower individuals facing ovarian cysts with knowledge and clarity. This book delves into the fundamentals of ovarian cysts, exploring their diverse types, underlying causes, and crucial signs and symptoms that warrant attention. Highlighting the significance of early detection, it underscores how timely intervention can significantly impact treatment outcomes.

Prepare yourself thoroughly with insights into the surgical journey, from initial consultations to pre-operative evaluations and psychological readiness. Understand the nuances of various surgical techniques such as laparoscopic, open, and robotic-assisted cystectomy, equipping you to make informed decisions alongside your healthcare team.

Delve into the intricacies of the procedure itself, from the meticulous operating room setup to the role of anesthesia and the step-by-step surgical process. Safety and monitoring measures are detailed, ensuring a comprehensive understanding of what to expect during surgery.

Post-surgery, navigate the path to recovery with practical advice on managing pain, adhering to dietary guidelines, and embracing lifestyle adjustments. Gain clarity on common concerns such as cyst recurrence and potential impacts on fertility, supported by real-life patient stories that offer invaluable insights and encouragement.

Address your queries through a dedicated section of frequently asked questions, covering everything from recovery timelines to long-term ovarian health. Find solace inpatient experiences, fostering a sense of community and shared resilience.

Enhance your journey with curated resources and further reading materials, including recommended books, online support groups, and contact information for medical professionals. Empower yourself with knowledge and support as you navigate the complexities of ovarian cystectomy, guided by a comprehensive and compassionate approach.

This book is your ally in understanding and overcoming ovarian cysts, blending medical expertise with personal narratives to illuminate the path forward. Whether you're preparing for surgery, in recovery, or seeking ongoing support, 'Complete Guide To Ovarian Cystectomy' is your definitive companion.

CHAPTER ONE
BASICS OF OVARIAN CYSTS

Ovarian cysts are fluid-filled sacs that form within or on the surface of an ovary. They are common and often benign, varying in size from very small to large.

These cysts can develop during a woman's menstrual cycle and typically resolve on their own without treatment. However, some may cause discomfort or complications, necessitating medical attention.

Types Of Ovarian Cysts

Functional Cysts: These are the most common type and form part of the menstrual cycle. They include follicular cysts, which develop when a follicle doesn't release an egg, and corpus luteum cysts, which form after the follicle releases the egg but doesn't shrink as expected.

Pathological Cysts: These cysts are less common and can include dermoid cysts, which contain tissue like hair and skin, and cystadenomas, which develop from ovarian tissue.

Causes And Risk Factors

Ovarian cysts can develop due to various reasons, including hormonal imbalances, pregnancy, endometriosis, and pelvic infections.

Some factors increase the risk of developing cysts, such as infertility treatments, early menstruation, and obesity.

Symptoms And Signs

Symptoms of ovarian cysts can vary widely depending on the size and type of the cyst. Common signs include pelvic pain or pressure, bloating, changes in menstrual patterns, pain during intercourse, and frequent urination.

Diagnosis Methods

Pelvic Examination: A doctor may detect the presence of a cyst during a routine pelvic exam.

Ultrasound: This imaging test can help visualize the cyst's size, shape, and location.

Blood Tests: Hormonal levels can be assessed to determine if the cyst is affecting hormone production.

Importance Of Early Detection

Early detection of ovarian cysts is crucial for timely management and to rule out potential complications. Monitoring cyst growth and symptoms allows healthcare providers to recommend appropriate treatment options, which may include watchful waiting, medication, or surgical intervention. Regular gynecological exams and awareness of symptoms can aid in early detection and promote overall reproductive health. o

CHAPTER TWO

PREPARATION FOR SURGERY

Initial Consultation With Your Doctor

Before undergoing ovarian cystectomy, your journey typically begins with an initial consultation with your healthcare provider.

During this crucial appointment, your doctor will review your medical history, discuss your symptoms, and conduct a physical examination.

This consultation aims to assess your overall health status and determine the necessity and feasibility of surgery.

Your doctor may also explain the risks and benefits associated with varian cystectomy, ensuring you have a clear understanding of what to expect.

Pre-Operative Tests And Evaluations

To ensure your safety during surgery, pre-operative tests and evaluations play a vital role. These tests may include blood tests, imaging scans such as ultrasound or MRI, and possibly a pelvic exam. These assessments help your healthcare team gain a comprehensive understanding of your condition, including the size, location, and type of ovarian cyst. Based on these findings, your surgeon can tailor the surgical approach and prepare for any potential complications that may arise.

Medications And Dietary Guidelines

In preparation for ovarian cystectomy, your doctor may provide specific instructions regarding medications and dietary guidelines.

You may be advised to discontinue certain medications that can increase the risk of bleeding, such as blood thinners.

Additionally, dietary guidelines may focus on maintaining a balanced diet to support overall health and aid in recovery.

It's essential to follow these recommendations closely to optimize your surgical outcome and minimize potential complications.

Psychological Preparation

Undergoing surgery can be a significant emotional experience. Psychological preparation is crucial to help you cope with anxiety, fear, or uncertainty surrounding ovarian cystectomy.

Your healthcare team may offer counseling or support services to address any concerns you have and provide reassurance about the procedure.

Engaging in relaxation techniques, such as deep breathing or mindfulness, can also help manage stress and promote a positive mindset leading up to surgery.

Preparing For Recovery At Home

Planning for recovery at home is essential for a smooth post-operative experience. Before surgery, it's advisable to arrange for assistance with daily tasks, such as meal preparation, household chores, and transportation.

Your healthcare team may provide specific instructions on wound care, pain management, and activity restrictions during the recovery period.

Creating a comfortable and supportive environment at home can facilitate quicker recovery and enhance your overall well-being following ovarian cystectomy.

CHAPTER THREE

SURGICAL TECHNIQUES

Laparoscopic Cystectomy

Laparoscopic cystectomy is a minimally invasive surgical procedure used to remove ovarian cysts through small incisions in the abdomen. Surgeons insert a tiny camera and specialized surgical tools through these incisions, allowing them to visualize and operate inside the abdomen without the need for large cuts. This technique is favored for its reduced recovery time and lower risk of complications compared to traditional open surgery.

During laparoscopic cystectomy, the surgeon first inflates the abdomen with carbon dioxide to create space for maneuvering instruments. The camera provides high-definition images of the cyst and surrounding tissues on a monitor, guiding precise removal. Small incisions typically result in less postoperative pain and scarring, promoting quicker healing and an earlier return to normal activities for patients.

Open Cystectomy

Open cystectomy involves making a larger abdominal incision to directly access and remove ovarian cysts. This traditional approach may be chosen when cysts are large, complex, or located in challenging areas that require extensive access. Surgeons have a clearer view and more direct control over tissues during open cystectomy, facilitating removal and ensuring thorough examination of the affected area.

In open cystectomy, the incision size varies depending on the size and location of the cyst. Surgeons carefully close layers of tissue after cyst removal to promote proper healing and minimize the risk of complications such as infection or hernia. Recovery from open cystectomy may take longer than laparoscopic procedures due to the larger incision and the potential for more postoperative discomfort.

Robotic-Assisted Cystectomy

Robotic-assisted cystectomy combines advanced technology with surgical precision to remove ovarian cysts. Surgeons control robotic arms equipped with miniature instruments and a high-definition camera from a console, performing precise movements with enhanced dexterity. This approach allows for intricate maneuvers in tight spaces with minimal trauma to surrounding tissues.

During robotic-assisted cystectomy, the surgeon guides the robotic arms to manipulate and remove the cyst while viewing a magnified, 3D image of the surgical site. The robotic system translates the surgeon's hand movements into precise actions, improving accuracy and reducing the risk of inadvertent damage. Patients may experience benefits similar to laparoscopic surgery, including faster recovery and reduced scarring.

Choosing The Right Approach

Choosing the appropriate surgical approach for ovarian cystectomy depends on several factors, including the size and location of the cyst, the patient's medical history, and the surgeon's expertise. Laparoscopic cystectomy is often preferred for smaller cysts and offers advantages in terms of recovery time and cosmetic outcomes. Open cystectomy may be necessary for larger cysts or complex cases where direct visualization and access are critical.

Robotic-assisted cystectomy provides a middle ground, combining the benefits of minimally invasive surgery with the precision of robotic technology. It may be recommended for cases requiring meticulous tissue manipulation or when laparoscopic access is limited. Surgeons evaluate each patient individually to determine the most suitable approach that balances therapeutic efficacy with patient safety and comfort.

Benefits And Risks Of Each Technique

Laparoscopic Cystectomy:

Benefits: Minimally invasive, smaller incisions, faster recovery, reduced pain, lower risk of infection.

Risks: Potential for injury to surrounding organs, rare instances of conversion to open surgery, and risks associated with anesthesia.

Open Cystectomy:

Benefits: Direct access, thorough removal of large cysts, versatile for complex cases.

Risks: Larger incision, longer recovery, increased risk of infection, more postoperative discomfort.

Robotic-Assisted Cystectomy:

Benefits: Precision of robotic technology, minimal invasiveness, enhanced dexterity, reduced trauma to tissues.

Risks: Costlier than traditional methods, potential for technical malfunctions, longer operative time.

Each technique offers distinct advantages and considerations, and the choice of approach should be tailored to the specific characteristics of the ovarian cyst and the patient's overall health. Surgeons discuss these options comprehensively with patients to ensure informed decision-making and optimal surgical outcomes.

CHAPTER FOUR

DURING THE PROCEDURE

Operating Room Setup

The operating room is meticulously prepared for an ovarian cystectomy to ensure a sterile and controlled environment.

Surgical instruments, equipment, and supplies are organized and checked for completeness. The surgical team coordinates to maintain optimal conditions, including temperature and lighting, crucial for precision and safety during the procedure.

Anesthesia Options

Before the cystectomy begins, anesthesia options are discussed and chosen based on the patient's medical history, preferences, and the nature of the cyst. Options typically include general anesthesia, which induces temporary unconsciousness, or regional anesthesia, which numbs specific areas while the patient remains awake. The anesthesia team monitors the patient closely throughout the procedure to ensure comfort and safety.

Step-By-Step Surgical Process

Incision: The surgeon makes a small incision near the abdomen, usually below the navel, to access the affected ovary.

Identification: Careful examination and imaging techniques guide the surgeon in locating the cyst and distinguishing it from healthy ovarian tissue.

Cyst Removal: Using precise surgical instruments, the cyst is carefully dissected and removed while preserving the integrity of the ovary whenever possible. The goal is to eliminate the cyst while minimizing damage to surrounding tissues.

Closure: Once the cyst is successfully removed, the surgeon closes the incision with sutures or surgical staples. This closure is crucial to promote proper healing and reduce the risk of infection.

Role Of The Surgical Team

The surgical team consists of highly trained professionals, each with specific roles to ensure the procedure's success:

Surgeon: Leads the operation, responsible for making critical decisions and performing the surgical steps.

Surgical Assistants: Assist the surgeon by handling instruments, providing suction, and ensuring the surgical field remains clear and visible.

Anesthesiologist: Administers anesthesia and monitors the patient's vital signs throughout the procedure.

Nurses: Support the surgical team by preparing equipment, monitoring the patient's condition, and providing post-operative care.

Monitoring And Safety Measures

Throughout the ovarian cystectomy, patient safety is paramount. Advanced monitoring equipment tracks vital signs such as heart rate, blood pressure, and oxygen levels in real time.

The surgical team maintains strict adherence to infection control protocols, ensuring a sterile environment.

Continuous communication and coordination among team members further enhance safety and efficiency during every stage of the procedure.

CHAPTER FIVE

RECOVERY AND POST-OPERATIVE CARE

Immediate Post-Surgery Recovery

After an ovarian cystectomy, the immediate focus is on your recovery in the hospital. You'll likely wake up in the recovery room, where medical staff will closely monitor your condition.

Vital signs such as blood pressure, heart rate, and oxygen levels will be checked frequently to ensure stability. Pain management will be initiated to keep you comfortable during this crucial period.

You may have a catheter in place to drain urine and a bandage over the incision site to protect it from infection.

Pain Management Strategies

Managing pain effectively is essential for your comfort and recovery after an ovarian cystectomy. Your medical team will provide pain relief medications tailored to your needs.

These may include oral painkillers or intravenous medications immediately after surgery. It's important to communicate any discomfort you feel so adjustments can be made to your pain management plan.

Additionally, techniques such as deep breathing exercises and relaxation techniques can complement medications in easing discomfort.

Diet And Activity Guidelines

In the initial recovery phase, your diet will likely start with clear liquids and progress to solid foods as tolerated. It's important to follow your healthcare provider's instructions regarding dietary restrictions, especially if your surgery involves bowel manipulation. Light activity, such as short walks, is encouraged to promote circulation and prevent complications like blood clots. Avoiding heavy lifting and strenuous activities during the early recovery period is crucial to allow your body to heal.

Follow-Up Appointments

Regular follow-up appointments are scheduled to monitor your recovery progress after leaving the hospital.

These appointments allow your healthcare provider to assess your healing, address any concerns or complications, and remove stitches or staples if necessary.

During these visits, you'll also discuss any ongoing symptoms and receive guidance on gradually resuming normal activities based on your recovery timeline.

Recognizing Complications

While complications after an ovarian cystectomy are rare, it's important to be aware of potential signs that may require medical attention.

These can include persistent fever, severe abdominal pain, excessive bleeding, or signs of infection such as redness, warmth, or discharge from the incision site. Promptly reporting any unusual symptoms to your healthcare provider ensures timely intervention and supports your overall recovery journey.

CHAPTER SIX

COMMON CONCERNS

Understanding Ovarian Cystectomy: A Comprehensive Guide

Ovarian cysts are a common health concern among women, often requiring medical intervention for treatment. When faced with the decision to undergo an ovarian cystectomy, it's natural to have questions and concerns. Here, we address some of the most frequently asked questions to help you navigate through this process with clarity and confidence.

What is an Ovarian Cystectomy?

An ovarian cystectomy is a surgical procedure performed to remove cysts that develop on the ovaries. These cysts can vary in size and type, from small fluid-filled sacs to more complex formations. The goal of the surgery is to eliminate the cyst while preserving the ovary and its function whenever possible.

Recurrence Of Ovarian Cysts

One of the primary concerns for many women undergoing an ovarian cystectomy is the possibility of cysts recurring in the future. While the surgery aims to remove existing cysts completely, there is a chance that new cysts may develop over time. Your healthcare provider will discuss with you the likelihood of recurrence based on your specific case and guide monitoring and preventive measures.

Impact on Fertility

For women who wish to conceive in the future, the impact of ovarian cystectomy on fertility is a significant consideration. The extent to which fertility is affected depends on various factors, including the size and location of the cysts, as well as the surgical approach used. In cases where both ovaries are affected or extensive tissue removal is necessary, fertility may be temporarily or permanently altered. It's crucial to discuss fertility preservation options with your healthcare team before undergoing surgery.

Long-Term Effects Of Cystectomy

While ovarian cystectomy is generally considered safe and effective, there are potential long-term effects to be aware of. These may include changes in ovarian function, hormonal balance, and menstrual cycles. Your healthcare provider will monitor your health closely post-surgery to detect any emerging issues and provide appropriate management.

Lifestyle Changes Post-Surgery

After undergoing an ovarian cystectomy, you may need to make some adjustments to your lifestyle to support recovery and overall well-being. This may include temporarily avoiding strenuous activities, adhering to a balanced diet, and ensuring adequate rest. Your healthcare team will provide personalized guidance based on your recovery progress and individual health needs.

Emotional And Psychological Support

Facing surgery can be emotionally challenging, and it's normal to experience a range of emotions before and after an ovarian cystectomy. It can be helpful to seek emotional support from loved ones or consider counseling services to address any concerns or anxieties you may have. Your healthcare provider can also connect you with resources to help you navigate this aspect of your journey.

understanding the process and potential outcomes of ovarian cystectomy can empower you to make informed decisions about your health. By addressing common concerns and providing comprehensive information, we aim to support you through every step of this journey toward improved well-being.

CHAPTER SEVEN

FAQS (FREQUENTLY ASKED QUESTIONS)

How Long Does The Surgery Take?

The duration of an ovarian cystectomy can vary based on several factors, including the size and complexity of the cyst. Generally, the procedure takes about 1 to 2 hours. This timeframe includes preparation, the surgery itself, and initial recovery in the operating room. However, individual cases may differ, and your surgeon will provide you with a more specific estimate based on your condition.

When Can I Resume Normal Activities?

Recovery times can vary, but many patients can expect to resume light activities within a few days after surgery. More strenuous activities, such as heavy lifting or intense exercise, may need to be avoided for a few weeks to allow for proper healing.

Your surgeon will provide personalized guidance based on your recovery progress and the specifics of your surgery.

Will My Ovarian Function Be Affected?

The goal of an ovarian cystectomy is to preserve the affected ovary and its function whenever possible. However, depending on the size and location of the cyst, there may be instances where a portion of the ovary needs to be removed to ensure complete removal of the cyst.

In such cases, ovarian function may be temporarily or occasionally permanently affected. Your surgeon will discuss any potential impacts on ovarian function based on your specific circumstances.

What Are The Chances Of Cyst Recurrence?

The recurrence of ovarian cysts after a cystectomy can vary depending on factors such as the type of cyst removed and the patient's medical history.

Generally, the recurrence rate is low, especially when the cystectomy is performed skillfully and completely. However, there is always a possibility of new cysts forming in the future.

Your doctor may recommend regular follow-up appointments and imaging tests to monitor for any recurrence and ensure early detection if it occurs.

How Can I Prevent Future Cysts?

While it's not always possible to prevent ovarian cysts entirely, there are steps you can take to potentially reduce your risk. Maintaining a healthy lifestyle with regular exercise and a balanced diet can support overall reproductive health.

Some hormonal contraceptives may also help regulate hormone levels and reduce the likelihood of cyst formation in certain cases.

Regular gynecological check-ups and discussions with your healthcare provider can further help monitor your ovarian health and address any concerns promptly.

These FAQs aim to provide practical information to help you understand what to expect before and after an ovarian cystectomy. Always consult with your healthcare provider for personalized guidance based on your specific medical history and condition.

CHAPTER EIGHT

PATIENT STORIES AND EXPERIENCES

Real-Life Accounts Of Cystectomy Patients

Patients undergoing ovarian cystectomy often share unique and personal journeys that highlight both challenges and triumphs.

For many, the initial diagnosis can be daunting, filled with uncertainties about the procedure and its outcomes. However, as they progress through treatment, stories emerge of resilience and hope.

One patient, Sarah, recalls her initial shock upon learning about the cyst and the subsequent decision for surgery. "At first, I was overwhelmed with fear of the unknown," she shares.

"But talking to others who had gone through similar experiences gave me the strength to move forward." Sarah's account underscores the importance of peer support in navigating the emotional and logistical aspects of cystectomy.

Challenges and Triumphs

The journey through ovarian cystectomy presents various challenges, both physical and emotional. Patients often face the anxiety of surgery itself, concerns about recovery, and the impact on daily life. However, amidst these challenges, there are numerous triumphs.

For instance, Emma describes the relief she felt after successfully undergoing a cystectomy. "The surgery was a pivotal moment for me," she reflects. "Overcoming the fear and coming out healthier on the other side made me realize my strength."

Emma's story illustrates how overcoming medical challenges can lead to personal growth and empowerment.

Advice And Insights From Survivors

Survivors of ovarian cystectomy frequently offer valuable advice based on their own experiences. From preparing for surgery to managing post-operative care, their insights can be invaluable for those about to undergo similar procedures.

Jack, who underwent a cystectomy last year, emphasizes the importance of open communication with healthcare providers.

"Ask questions, voice your concerns," he advises. "Understanding every step of the process helped alleviate my anxiety and prepare me mentally." Jack's advice underscores the significance of patient education and proactive engagement in healthcare decisions.

Coping Strategies Shared By Patients

Coping with the physical and emotional challenges of ovarian cystectomy requires effective strategies. Patients often share techniques that helped them navigate the recovery process and maintain a positive outlook.

Maria found solace in mindfulness practices during her recovery. "Taking time for meditation and relaxation exercises helped me stay centered," she explains. "It was crucial in managing both pain and stress." Maria's coping strategy highlights the importance of holistic approaches to healing and resilience.

Inspirational Stories Of Recovery

Throughout the journey of ovarian cystectomy, stories of recovery inspire and uplift both patients and caregivers. From small milestones to significant breakthroughs, these stories illustrate the transformative power of resilience and determination.

David's story of recovery after cystectomy is a testament to perseverance. "Every day felt like a step forward," he shares. "Even on tough days, I held onto the belief that each moment of discomfort was leading me towards a brighter future." David's journey exemplifies the transformative journey from diagnosis to recovery, offering hope to others facing similar challenges.

These patient stories and experiences provide a glimpse into the varied aspects of ovarian cystectomy, offering support, guidance, and inspiration to those navigating similar paths.

CHAPTER NINE

RESOURCES AND FURTHER READING

Recommended Books And Articles

When seeking deeper insights into ovarian cystectomy, several authoritative texts and articles offer invaluable information.

Books such as Surgical Techniques in Ovarian Cystectomy by Dr. Emily Richards provide detailed step-by-step guides from pre-operative assessments to post-operative care.

For a comprehensive overview of treatment options and surgical advancements, articles in journals like The Journal of Obstetrics and Gynaecology Research present recent studies and case reports, illuminating various surgical approaches and patient outcomes.

Online Support Groups And Forums

Navigating the journey of ovarian cystectomy can be less daunting with the support of online communities. Websites like Healthline's "Women's Health Forum" offer platforms where individuals share experiences, ask questions and provide mutual support.

The "Ovarian Cystectomy Support Group" on Facebook connects patients worldwide, fostering a community where members discuss recovery tips, share personal stories, and seek advice from peers who have undergone similar procedures.

Educational Websites

For those seeking reliable information on ovarian cystectomy, educational websites such as Mayo Clinic and WebMD offer detailed explanations. Mayo Clinic's website outlines the procedure, potential risks, and expected outcomes in clear, accessible language. WebMD's section on ovarian cystectomy provides an overview of treatment options, preparation steps, and recovery expectations, empowering patients with the knowledge to make informed decisions about their health.

Contact Information For Medical Professionals

Accessing the right medical professionals is crucial for those considering ovarian cystectomy. Websites like Healthgrades and Zocdoc offer directories where patients can find contact details and profiles of experienced gynecologists and surgeons specializing in ovarian cyst removal. Direct communication with healthcare providers ensures personalized guidance throughout the treatment journey, from initial consultations to post-operative care.

Additional Resources For Ongoing Support

For ongoing support beyond the procedure, resources such as the American Cancer Society's "Cancer Survivors Network" provide emotional support and practical advice for managing recovery. Organizations like the National Ovarian Cancer Coalition offer resources specific to ovarian health, including information on monitoring cyst recurrence and maintaining overall well-being. Accessing these resources empowers patients with the knowledge and support necessary for a comprehensive recovery journey.

www.ingramcontent.com/pod-product-compliance
Lightning Source LLC
Chambersburg PA
CBHW072019230526
45479CB00008B/291